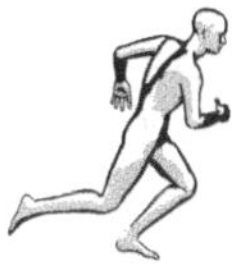

RUN! RUN! RUN!
WORKOUT PLANNER

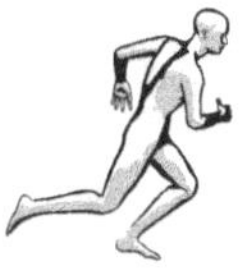

DATE:

	DISTANCE	TIME	HR
DAY 1			
DAY 2			
DAY 3			
DAY 4			
DAY 5			

NOTES:

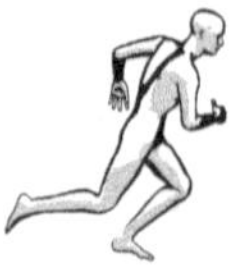

RUN! RUN! RUN!

WORKOUT PLANNER

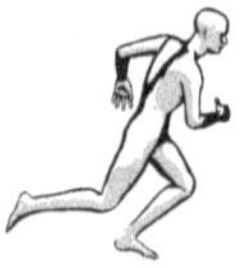

DATE:

	DISTANCE	TIME	HR
DAY 1			
DAY 2			
DAY 3			
DAY 4			
DAY 5			

NOTES:

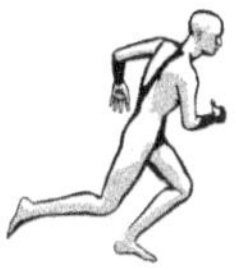

RUN! RUN! RUN!

WORKOUT PLANNER

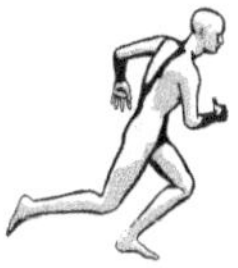

DATE:

	DISTANCE	TIME	HR
DAY 1			
DAY 2			
DAY 3			
DAY 4			
DAY 5			

NOTES:

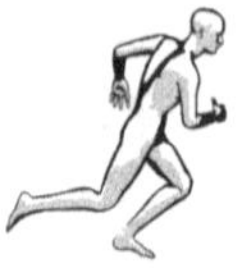

RUN! RUN! RUN!
WORKOUT PLANNER

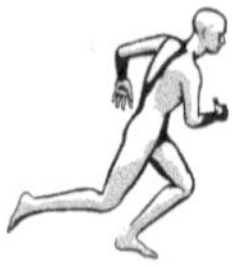

DATE:

	DISTANCE	TIME	HR
DAY 1			
DAY 2			
DAY 3			
DAY 4			
DAY 5			

NOTES:

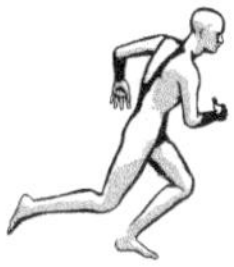

RUN! RUN! RUN!
WORKOUT PLANNER

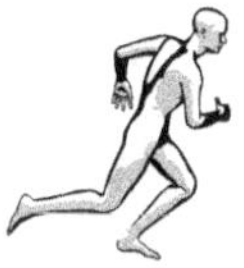

DATE:

	DISTANCE	TIME	HR
DAY 1			
DAY 2			
DAY 3			
DAY 4			
DAY 5			

NOTES:

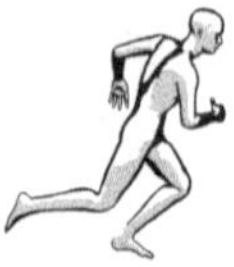

RUN! RUN! RUN!
WORKOUT PLANNER

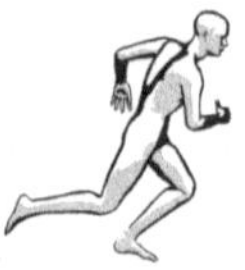

DATE:

	DISTANCE	TIME	HR
DAY 1			
DAY 2			
DAY 3			
DAY 4			
DAY 5			

NOTES:

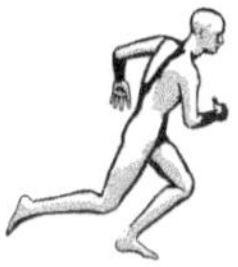

RUN! RUN! RUN!
WORKOUT PLANNER

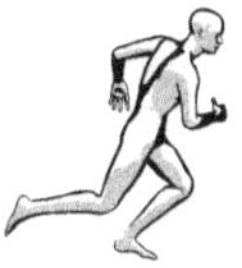

DATE:

	DISTANCE	TIME	HR
DAY 1			
DAY 2			
DAY 3			
DAY 4			
DAY 5			

NOTES:

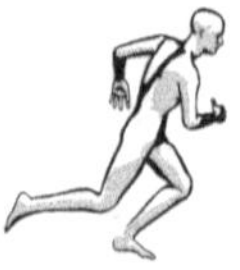

RUN! RUN! RUN!

WORKOUT PLANNER

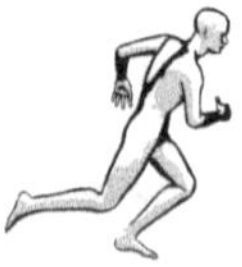

DATE:

	DISTANCE	TIME	HR
DAY 1			
DAY 2			
DAY 3			
DAY 4			
DAY 5			

NOTES:

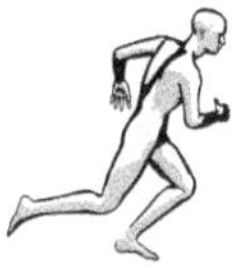

RUN! RUN! RUN!
WORKOUT PLANNER

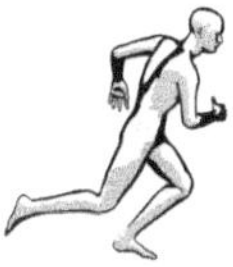

DATE:

	DISTANCE	TIME	HR
DAY 1			
DAY 2			
DAY 3			
DAY 4			
DAY 5			

NOTES:

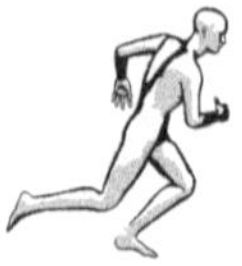

RUN! RUN! RUN!

WORKOUT PLANNER

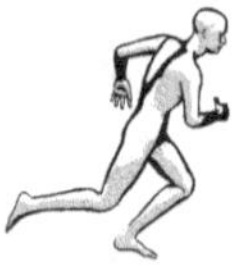

DATE:

	DISTANCE	TIME	HR
DAY 1			
DAY 2			
DAY 3			
DAY 4			
DAY 5			

NOTES:

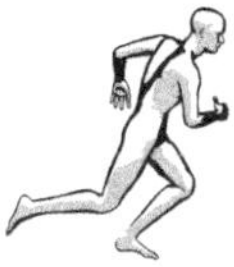

RUN! RUN! RUN!
WORKOUT PLANNER

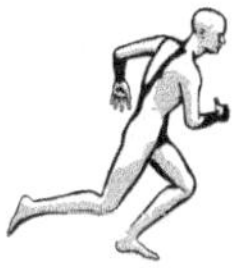

DATE:

	DISTANCE	TIME	HR
DAY 1			
DAY 2			
DAY 3			
DAY 4			
DAY 5			

NOTES:

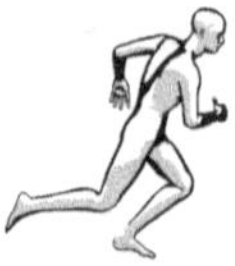

RUN! RUN! RUN!
WORKOUT PLANNER

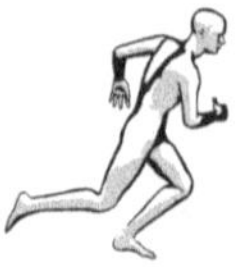

DATE:

	DISTANCE	TIME	HR
DAY 1			
DAY 2			
DAY 3			
DAY 4			
DAY 5			

NOTES:

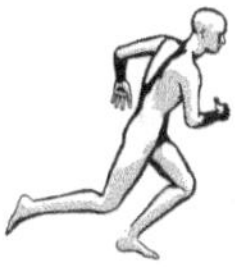

RUN! RUN! RUN!
WORKOUT PLANNER

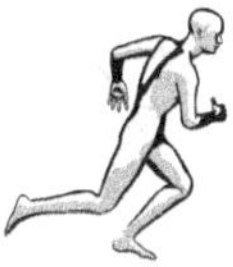

DATE:

	DISTANCE	TIME	HR
DAY 1			
DAY 2			
DAY 3			
DAY 4			
DAY 5			

NOTES:

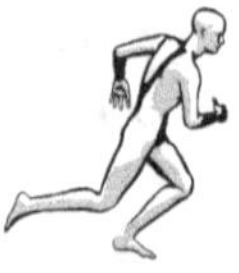

RUN! RUN! RUN!

WORKOUT PLANNER

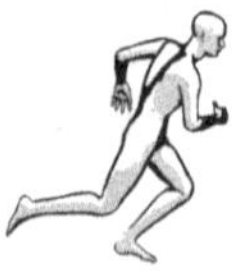

DATE:

	DISTANCE	TIME	HR
DAY 1			
DAY 2			
DAY 3			
DAY 4			
DAY 5			

NOTES:

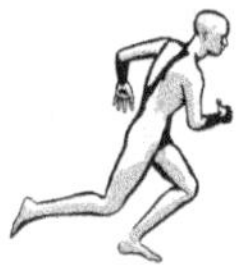

RUN! RUN! RUN!
WORKOUT PLANNER

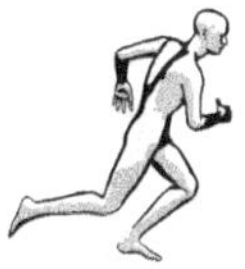

DATE:

	DISTANCE	TIME	HR
DAY 1			
DAY 2			
DAY 3			
DAY 4			
DAY 5			

NOTES:

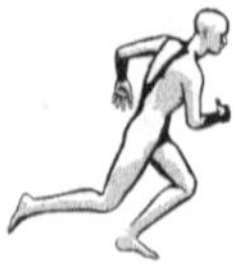

RUN! RUN! RUN!
WORKOUT PLANNER

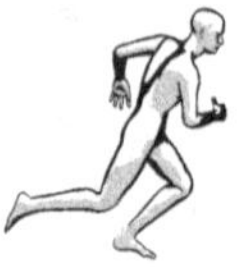

DATE:

	DISTANCE	TIME	HR
DAY 1			
DAY 2			
DAY 3			
DAY 4			
DAY 5			

NOTES:

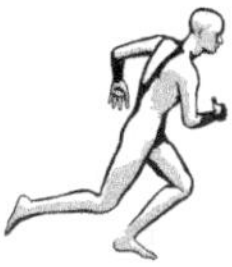

RUN! RUN! RUN!
WORKOUT PLANNER

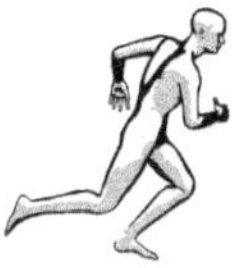

DATE:

	DISTANCE	TIME	HR
DAY 1			
DAY 2			
DAY 3			
DAY 4			
DAY 5			

NOTES:

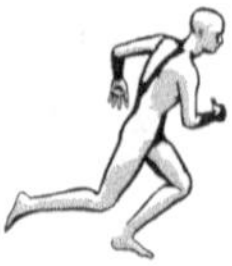

RUN! RUN! RUN!

WORKOUT PLANNER

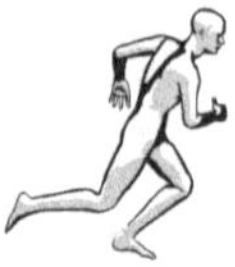

DATE:

	DISTANCE	TIME	HR
DAY 1			
DAY 2			
DAY 3			
DAY 4			
DAY 5			

NOTES:

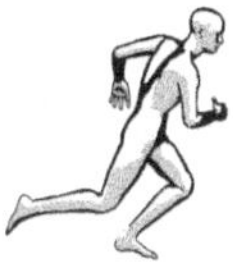

RUN! RUN! RUN!
WORKOUT PLANNER

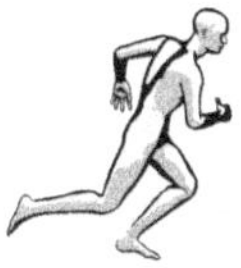

DATE:

	DISTANCE	TIME	HR
DAY 1			
DAY 2			
DAY 3			
DAY 4			
DAY 5			

NOTES:

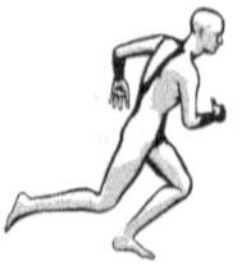

RUN! RUN! RUN!
WORKOUT PLANNER

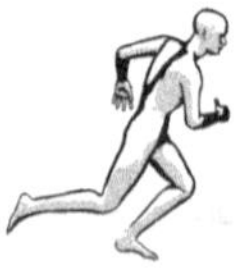

DATE:

	DISTANCE	TIME	HR
DAY 1			
DAY 2			
DAY 3			
DAY 4			
DAY 5			

NOTES:

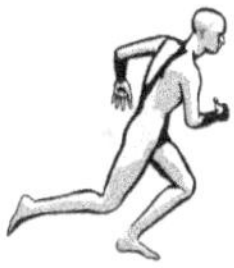

RUN! RUN! RUN!
WORKOUT PLANNER

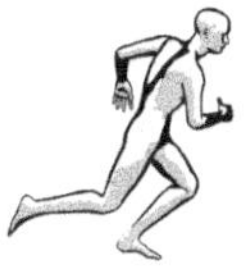

DATE:

	DISTANCE	TIME	HR
DAY 1			
DAY 2			
DAY 3			
DAY 4			
DAY 5			

NOTES:

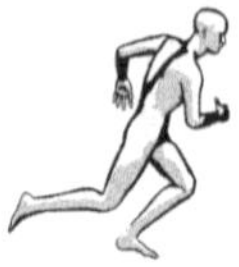

RUN! RUN! RUN!
WORKOUT PLANNER

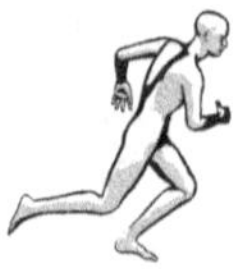

DATE:

	DISTANCE	TIME	HR
DAY 1			
DAY 2			
DAY 3			
DAY 4			
DAY 5			

NOTES:

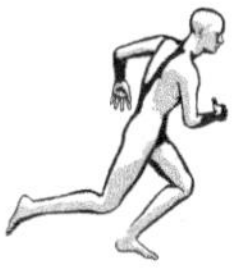

RUN! RUN! RUN!
WORKOUT PLANNER

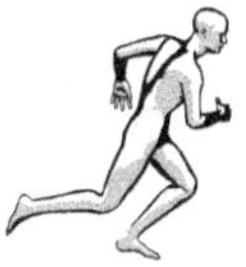

DATE:

	DISTANCE	TIME	HR
DAY 1			
DAY 2			
DAY 3			
DAY 4			
DAY 5			

NOTES:

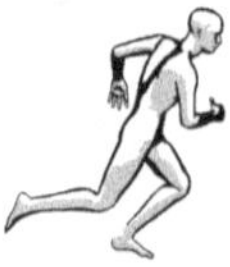

RUN! RUN! RUN!
WORKOUT PLANNER

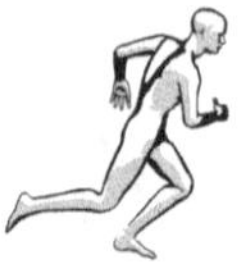

DATE:

	DISTANCE	TIME	HR
DAY 1			
DAY 2			
DAY 3			
DAY 4			
DAY 5			

NOTES:

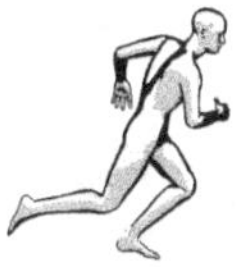

RUN! RUN! RUN!
WORKOUT PLANNER

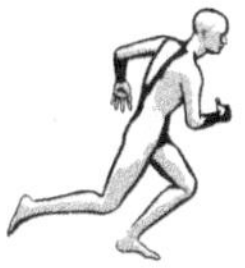

DATE:

	DISTANCE	TIME	HR
DAY 1			
DAY 2			
DAY 3			
DAY 4			
DAY 5			

NOTES:

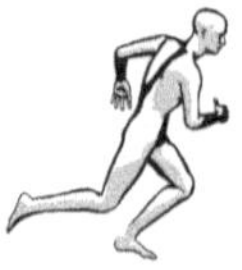

RUN! RUN! RUN!
WORKOUT PLANNER

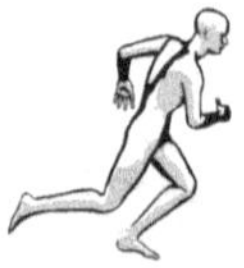

DATE:

	DISTANCE	TIME	HR
DAY 1			
DAY 2			
DAY 3			
DAY 4			
DAY 5			

NOTES:

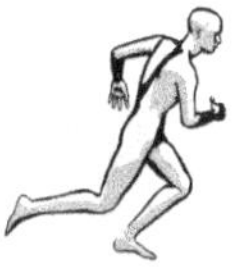

RUN! RUN! RUN!
WORKOUT PLANNER

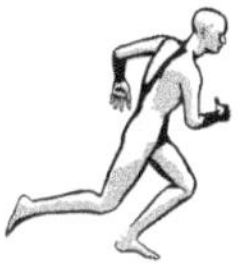

DATE:

	DISTANCE	TIME	HR
DAY 1			
DAY 2			
DAY 3			
DAY 4			
DAY 5			

NOTES:

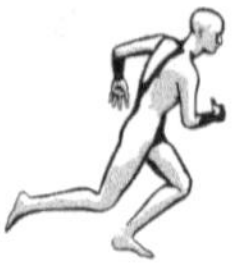

RUN! RUN! RUN!
WORKOUT PLANNER

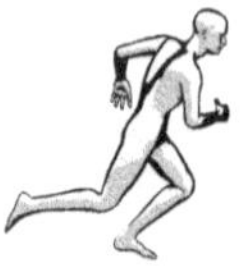

DATE:

DISTANCE	TIME	HR
DAY 1		
DAY 2		
DAY 3		
DAY 4		
DAY 5		

NOTES:

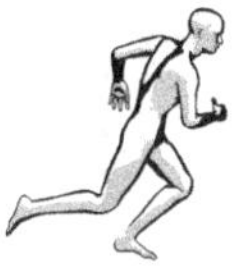

RUN! RUN! RUN!
WORKOUT PLANNER

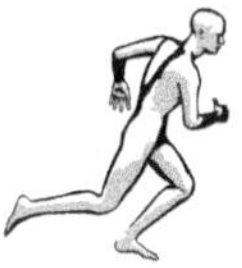

DATE:

	DISTANCE	TIME	HR
DAY 1			
DAY 2			
DAY 3			
DAY 4			
DAY 5			

NOTES:

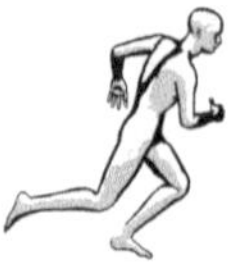

RUN! RUN! RUN!
WORKOUT PLANNER

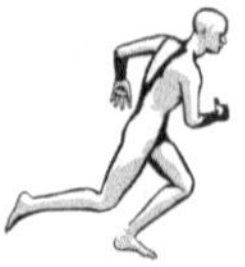

DATE:

	DISTANCE	TIME	HR
DAY 1			
DAY 2			
DAY 3			
DAY 4			
DAY 5			

NOTES:

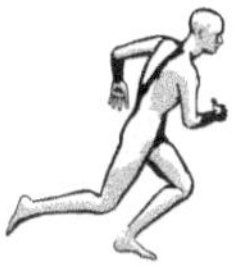

RUN! RUN! RUN!
WORKOUT PLANNER

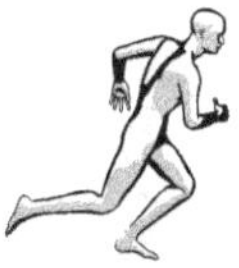

DATE:

	DISTANCE	TIME	HR
DAY 1			
DAY 2			
DAY 3			
DAY 4			
DAY 5			

NOTES:

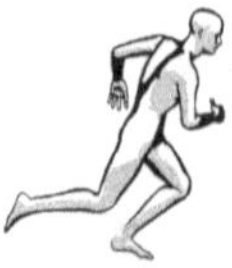

RUN! RUN! RUN!

WORKOUT PLANNER

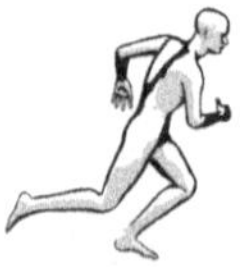

DATE:

	DISTANCE	TIME	HR
DAY 1			
DAY 2			
DAY 3			
DAY 4			
DAY 5			

NOTES:

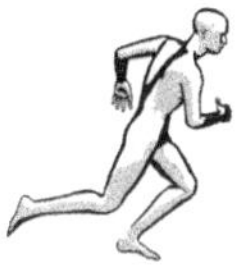

RUN! RUN! RUN!
WORKOUT PLANNER

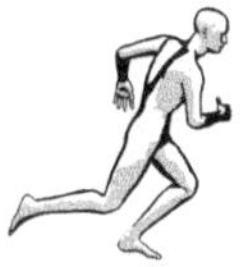

DATE:

	DISTANCE	TIME	HR
DAY 1			
DAY 2			
DAY 3			
DAY 4			
DAY 5			

NOTES:

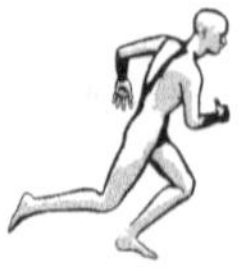

RUN! RUN! RUN!
WORKOUT PLANNER

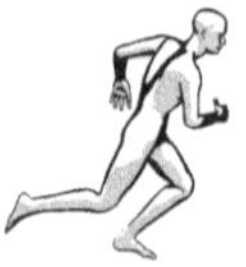

DATE:

	DISTANCE	TIME	HR
DAY 1			
DAY 2			
DAY 3			
DAY 4			
DAY 5			

NOTES:

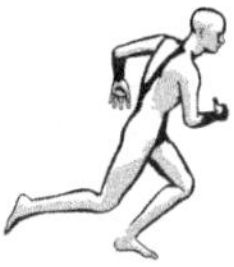

RUN! RUN! RUN!

WORKOUT PLANNER

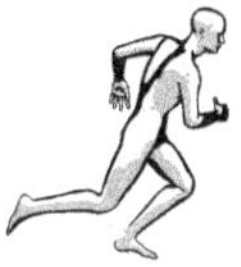

DATE:

	DISTANCE	TIME	HR
DAY 1			
DAY 2			
DAY 3			
DAY 4			
DAY 5			

NOTES:

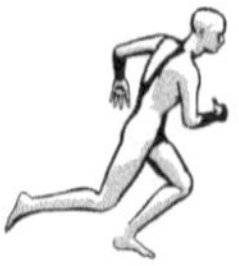

RUN! RUN! RUN!

WORKOUT PLANNER

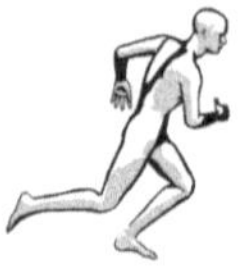

DATE:

	DISTANCE	TIME	HR
DAY 1			
DAY 2			
DAY 3			
DAY 4			
DAY 5			

NOTES:

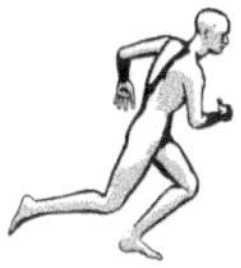

RUN! RUN! RUN!
WORKOUT PLANNER

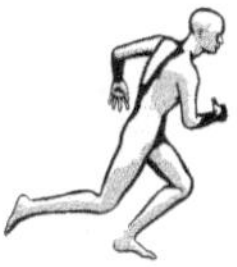

DATE:

	DISTANCE	TIME	HR
DAY 1			
DAY 2			
DAY 3			
DAY 4			
DAY 5			

NOTES:

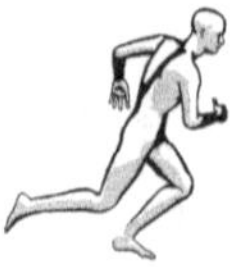

RUN! RUN! RUN!
WORKOUT PLANNER

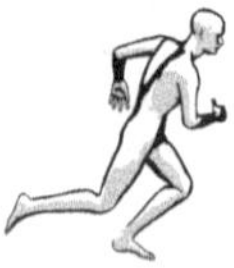

DATE:

	DISTANCE	TIME	HR
DAY 1			
DAY 2			
DAY 3			
DAY 4			
DAY 5			

NOTES:

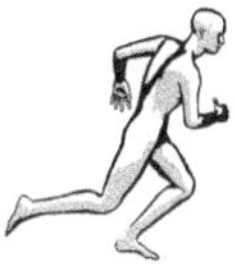

RUN! RUN! RUN!
WORKOUT PLANNER

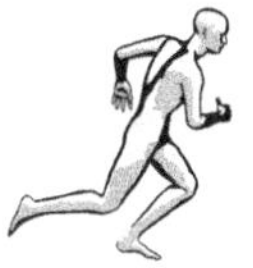

DATE:

	DISTANCE	TIME	HR
DAY 1			
DAY 2			
DAY 3			
DAY 4			
DAY 5			

NOTES:

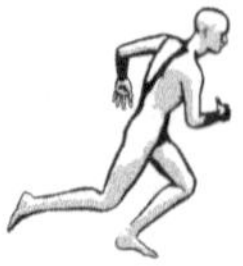

RUN! RUN! RUN!

WORKOUT PLANNER

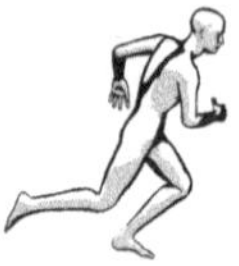

DATE:

	DISTANCE	TIME	HR
DAY 1			
DAY 2			
DAY 3			
DAY 4			
DAY 5			

NOTES:

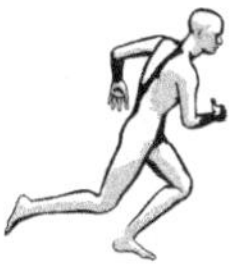

RUN! RUN! RUN!
WORKOUT PLANNER

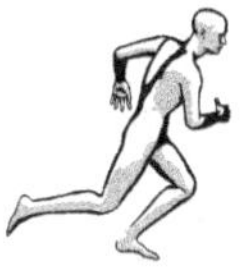

DATE:

	DISTANCE	TIME	HR
DAY 1			
DAY 2			
DAY 3			
DAY 4			
DAY 5			

NOTES:

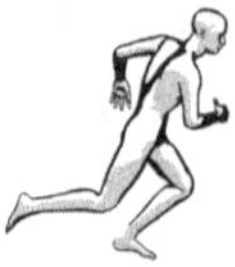

RUN! RUN! RUN!
WORKOUT PLANNER

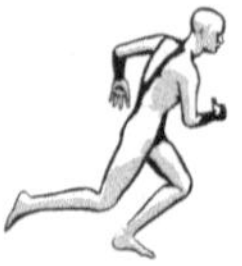

DATE:

	DISTANCE	TIME	HR
DAY 1			
DAY 2			
DAY 3			
DAY 4			
DAY 5			

NOTES:

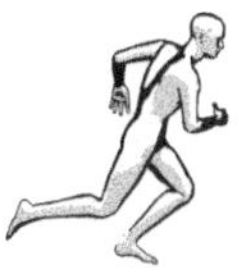

RUN! RUN! RUN!
WORKOUT PLANNER

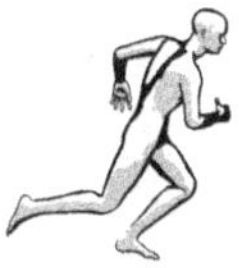

DATE:

	DISTANCE	TIME	HR
DAY 1			
DAY 2			
DAY 3			
DAY 4			
DAY 5			

NOTES:

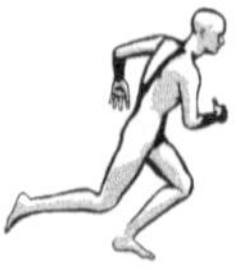

RUN! RUN! RUN!

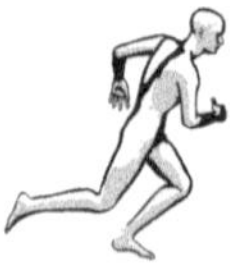

WORKOUT PLANNER

DATE:

	DISTANCE	TIME	HR
DAY 1			
DAY 2			
DAY 3			
DAY 4			
DAY 5			

NOTES:

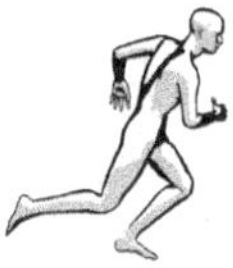

RUN! RUN! RUN!
WORKOUT PLANNER

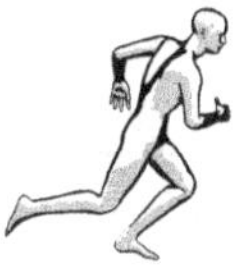

DATE:

	DISTANCE	TIME	HR
DAY 1			
DAY 2			
DAY 3			
DAY 4			
DAY 5			

NOTES:

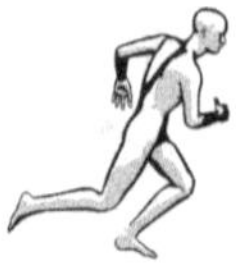

RUN! RUN! RUN!

WORKOUT PLANNER

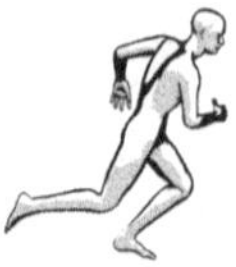

DATE:

	DISTANCE	TIME	HR
DAY 1			
DAY 2			
DAY 3			
DAY 4			
DAY 5			

NOTES:

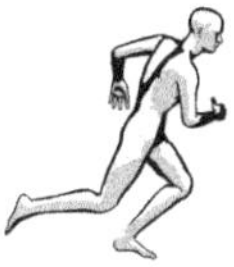

RUN! RUN! RUN!
WORKOUT PLANNER

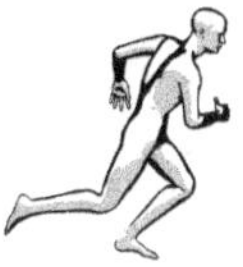

DATE:

	DISTANCE	TIME	HR
DAY 1			
DAY 2			
DAY 3			
DAY 4			
DAY 5			

NOTES:

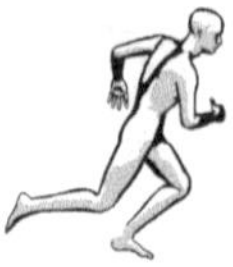

RUN! RUN! RUN!
WORKOUT PLANNER

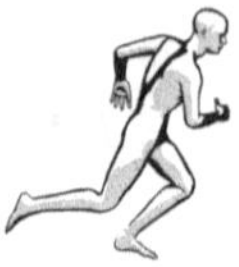

DATE:

	DISTANCE	TIME	HR
DAY 1			
DAY 2			
DAY 3			
DAY 4			
DAY 5			

NOTES:

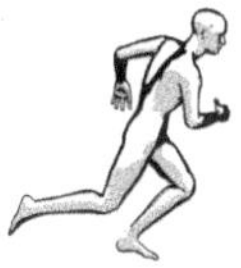

RUN! RUN! RUN!

WORKOUT PLANNER

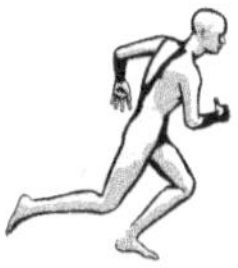

DATE:

	DISTANCE	TIME	HR
DAY 1			
DAY 2			
DAY 3			
DAY 4			
DAY 5			

NOTES:

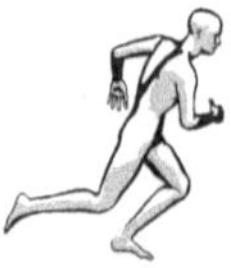

RUN! RUN! RUN!
WORKOUT PLANNER

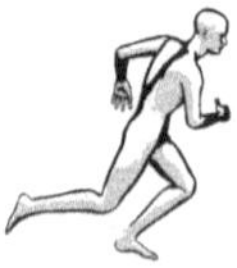

DATE:

	DISTANCE	TIME	HR
DAY 1			
DAY 2			
DAY 3			
DAY 4			
DAY 5			

NOTES:

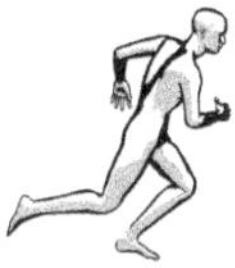

RUN! RUN! RUN!
WORKOUT PLANNER

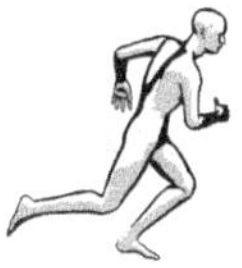

DATE:

	DISTANCE	TIME	HR
DAY 1			
DAY 2			
DAY 3			
DAY 4			
DAY 5			

NOTES:

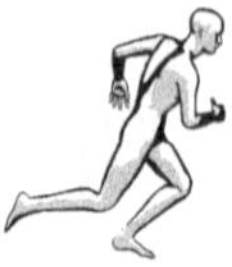

RUN! RUN! RUN!
WORKOUT PLANNER

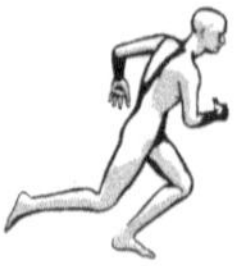

DATE:

	DISTANCE	TIME	HR
DAY 1			
DAY 2			
DAY 3			
DAY 4			
DAY 5			

NOTES:

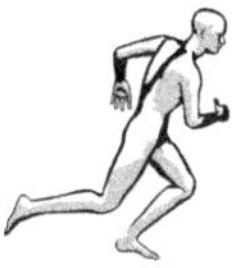

RUN! RUN! RUN!
WORKOUT PLANNER

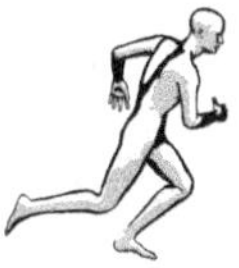

DATE:

	DISTANCE	TIME	HR
DAY 1			
DAY 2			
DAY 3			
DAY 4			
DAY 5			

NOTES:

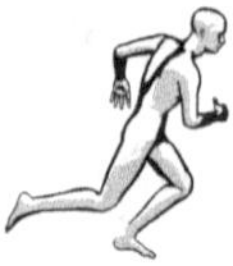

RUN! RUN! RUN!
WORKOUT PLANNER

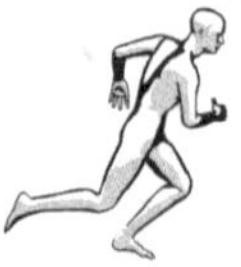

DATE:

	DISTANCE	TIME	HR
DAY 1			
DAY 2			
DAY 3			
DAY 4			
DAY 5			

NOTES:

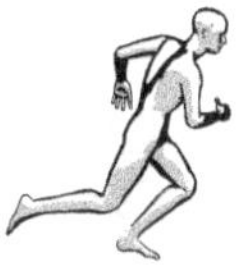

RUN! RUN! RUN!
WORKOUT PLANNER

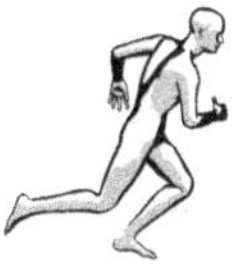

DATE:

	DISTANCE	TIME	HR
DAY 1			
DAY 2			
DAY 3			
DAY 4			
DAY 5			

NOTES:

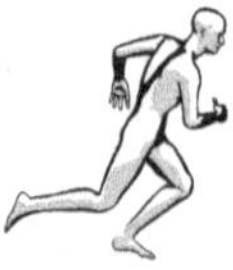

RUN! RUN! RUN!
WORKOUT PLANNER

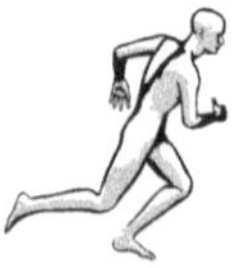

DATE:

	DISTANCE	TIME	HR
DAY 1			
DAY 2			
DAY 3			
DAY 4			
DAY 5			

NOTES:

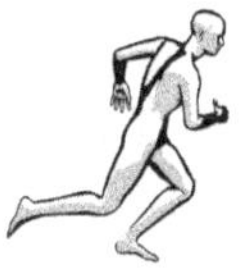

RUN! RUN! RUN!
WORKOUT PLANNER

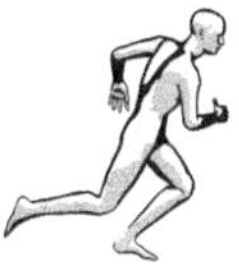

DATE:

	DISTANCE	TIME	HR
DAY 1			
DAY 2			
DAY 3			
DAY 4			
DAY 5			

NOTES:

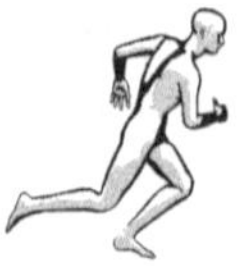

RUN! RUN! RUN!
WORKOUT PLANNER

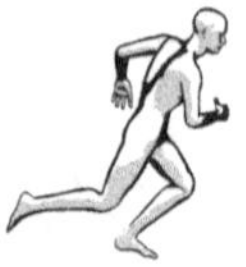

DATE:

	DISTANCE	TIME	HR
DAY 1			
DAY 2			
DAY 3			
DAY 4			
DAY 5			

NOTES:

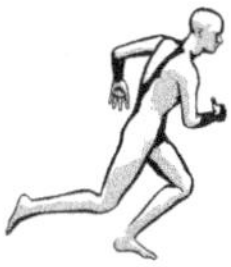

RUN! RUN! RUN!
WORKOUT PLANNER

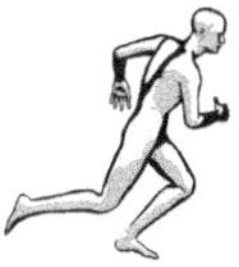

DATE:

	DISTANCE	TIME	HR
DAY 1			
DAY 2			
DAY 3			
DAY 4			
DAY 5			

NOTES:

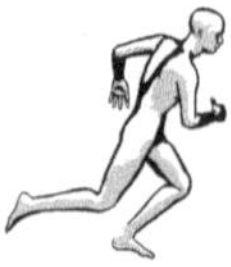

RUN! RUN! RUN!
WORKOUT PLANNER

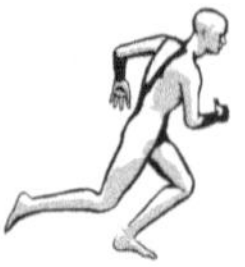

DATE:

	DISTANCE	TIME	HR
DAY 1			
DAY 2			
DAY 3			
DAY 4			
DAY 5			

NOTES:

www.ingramcontent.com/pod-product-compliance
Lightning Source LLC
Chambersburg PA
CBHW072118280526
45788CB00006B/2544
* 9 7 8 1 0 8 8 4 2 9 5 3 2 *